Hi, Momm

Here I Come!

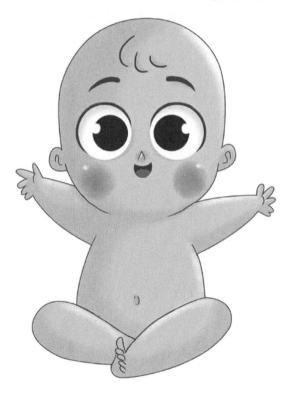

Mia Lenz

I hope you will enjoy reading and experiencing this book!
Please recommend this book to others or leave a positive review on Amazon if you enjoyed this book!

ISBN : 9798759601135

This book was printed on acid-free paper with chlorine-free ink.

Author: Mia Lenz
Translation: Alexandra Vaughn
Publisher: Tobias Bogdanov

Dear Mommy-to-be,

Congratulations to the little miracle that is growing inside your belly! The next few months will be incredibly exciting and full of change. Pregnancy is a very special time for you and your child. Cherish this time as much as you can, even if it seems difficult at times.

The greatest challenge that lies ahead is not yours, but your baby's! In just nine months, your baby will develop from a fertilized egg to a complete human being! The following pages will tell you about the many things your baby will experience during the next 40 weeks – and what it thinks about all of this excitement.

I hope you will enjoy this book, and I wish you and your baby a healthy and joyful pregnancy.

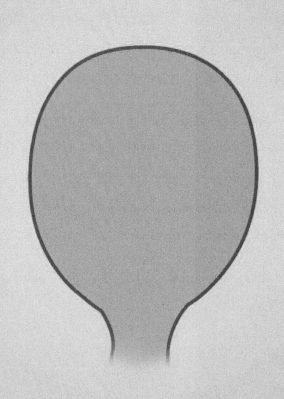

Cleaning up my new home

Hi, Mommy! I have great news for you — I have decided to move in with you! Unfortunately, fertilization was not successful during your last cycle, but as the saying goes: "another month, another chance".

Dear Mommy, I am not here just yet. However, it looks like I will surprise you very soon. To ensure that your uterus will be a cozy home for me, we need to tidy up a little bit. The uterine lining that grew during your last cycle has to be cleaned out. Once that is accomplished, the uterine lining will thicken once more — just for me!

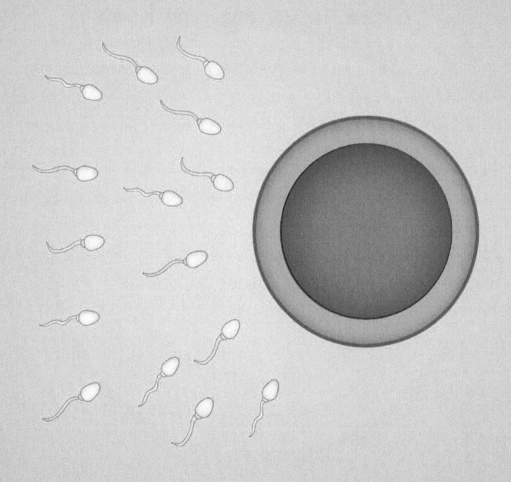

Who will get there first?

Oh, things are getting serious now! Ovulation has occurred.

I am still a sperm cell, but I am on my way to inspect my new home. They must have been joking when they said: "Just for you"! There are millions of other interested applicants who are trying to snag this apartment. Well, they do not stand a chance!

Phew, I really have to hurry if I want to be faster than the rest! It is quite far, and the conditions are not that friendly. My persistence pays off! I have reached the fallopian tube, and now I can see it: a large egg. It is love at first sight!

And I am the first one here! Nothing can stop me now! Mommy, you are stuck with me now!

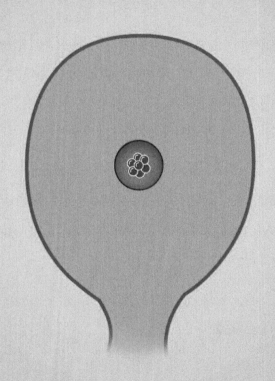

I am moving in

Well, I successfully completed the main challenge! The egg and sperm cells have combined, and cell division can begin. The color of my eyes, my sex, and my height are already predetermined. I am excited to find out what I will look like!

A short, but very important journey lies ahead. Fertilization occurred in the fallopian tube, and now I have to make my way to the uterus. There is not enough room to grow in the fallopian tube. I need lots of space because I want to grow big and strong.

I will arrive there by the end of the third week. This will be my home for the next few months, and I am making myself comfortable. Although a lot has happened already, Mommy probably has not even noticed my presence yet. Haha, I promise that this will change soon!

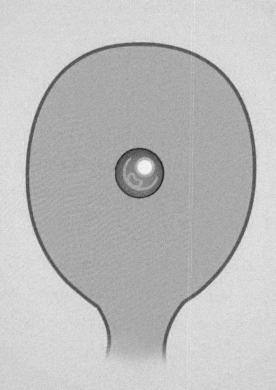

The move was successful

I have finally moved in. The placenta, yolk, and amniotic sac are developing because I need to be cared for as long as I live here!

Usually, the old uterine lining would be discharged right now, but everything is different this month! Finally, a guest who appreciates this comfortable interior has arrived – me!

My Mommy and Daddy cannot see me on the ultrasound, because I am only about 0.04 inches tall. I will keep an eye on them to see what they are up to!

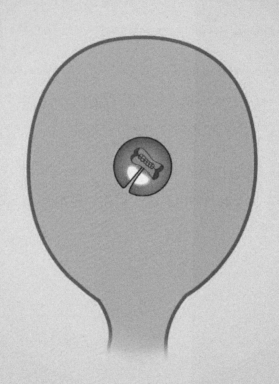

Announcing my arrival

Mommy may have started to notice my presence by now. If she has been longing for a child and decides to take an early pregnancy test, she will be very excited. What a beautiful surprise! Mom and Dad will be incredibly happy.

A lot of things are happening to me during the 5th week! I am still tiny and barely visible to the naked eye, but my organs are already developing. Heart, lungs, blood vessels, connective tissue, and sex organs are starting to develop. I have everything that a human needs! And that is what I want to be one day!

I still do not really look like a human. Instead, I resemble an oval disc, but I am confident that this will change soon!

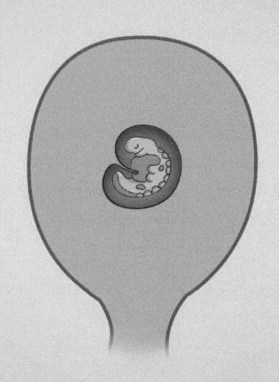

My Heart is beating

What is that? I am so excited because I heard a thump. That must be my heartbeat! It starts out with a pretty slow rhythm, but it will accelerate to a frequency of about 100 to 120 beats per minute very soon. My heart beats about twice as fast as my Mommy's!

Speaking of speed: I am experiencing a developmental spurt during the 6th week. I no longer look like a tiny disc. I look like a little worm. If you have a vivid imagination, you can tell that I will be a real baby one day! And there's more: my mouth, jaw, and vocal cords are starting to develop. My kidneys and stomach are starting to work.

I am now between 0.08 and 0.15 inches long. Mommy can see me for the very first time during the ultrasound. Hi, Mommy! Here I am!

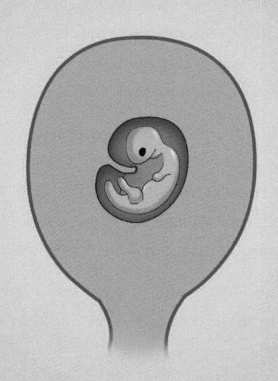

I have a face

Wow! My head is suddenly growing really fast, and lots of dimples and bumps have appeared on it! I wonder what those will turn into? I believe that the little dimples on the side of my head could turn into ears. The little bump in the middle of my face is probably going to be my nose.

Something is missing. I already have a mouth, but I would like to see things. Ah, luckily my eyes are starting to develop as well!

Another exciting thing is happening. Although it is already determined whether I will be a boy or a girl, both features developed at first. That has changed now. The sex characteristics are forming, but Mommy and Daddy will have to wait a little bit longer before they find out whether they will have a son or a daughter. I won't tell them just yet!

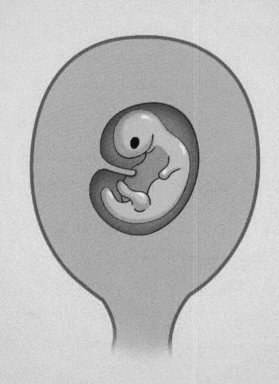

My intestines are growing quickly

Growth is a tricky thing. My intestines are growing rapidly, and they no longer fit into my belly. A loop of my intestines now protrudes into the umbilical cord, and this causes an umbilical hernia. Don't worry, it's not dangerous for me at all!

The growth of my organs is keeping me busy. My liver looks like a small bulge between my heart and the umbilical cord. You may think that all of these changes could make me nervous, but I feel comfortable and protected with my Mommy. I gently float around in the amniotic sac, and it shields me from noise and pressure.

I still require only a few ounces of amniotic fluid to float, but I will soon need a much larger amount if I continue to grow at this rate!

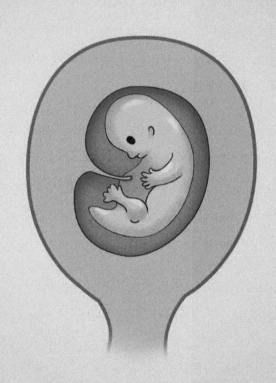

I have fingers and toes

I am transforming from a little worm into a baby. I have noticed that tiny fingers and toes are developing on my hands and feet. I wonder what I will be able to do with them in the future?

I measure around 0.5 to 1 inch. My eyes are still located at the side of my head, and that makes me look like a little alien. Nonetheless, nobody can deny that I will be a human one day. I will probably be very beautiful, too! I wonder if I will take after Mommy or Daddy.

Although I am still tiny, my organs are almost fully developed. My liver is already working. I still don't take up much room in Mommy's belly, and her pants still fit. I think her breasts have grown. I don't care too much about that, but Daddy seems to be very happy about it.

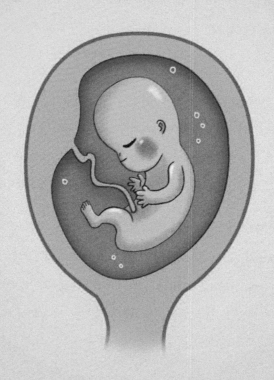

My taste buds are developing

Everything is here! I have arms, legs, knees, elbows, fingers, and toes.

I still have webbed toes and fingers, but the skin is gradually disappearing. My senses are improving, and I can suddenly taste things. I have learned a new skill: I can open and close my mouth! Of course, I am practicing this new ability diligently.

I can move around much better. I cannot perform a somersault in Mommy's belly yet, but I am sure I will get there one day. My movements are still very gentle. Mommy receives lots of compliments because she is glowing.

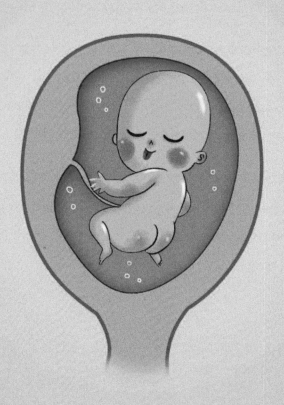

I am exercising a lot

I am much more active and have started to do water aerobics inside the amniotic sac. It is supposed to train my muscles and nerves, but I mainly do it because it is so much fun. My soft skin is starting to thicken, and a soft coat of hair covers my entire body — just like a little hamster. The nails on my fingers and toes are growing as well.

I like to show off my acrobatic skills on the ultrasound. I want Mommy and Daddy to see what I can do! What is Mommy's doctor looking at all the time? I think he is still trying to figure out if I will be a boy or a girl, but that's none of his business! I'll just show him my newly developed bootie.

Mommy needs to use the restroom frequently. I think that might be my fault because I am putting some pressure on her bladder.

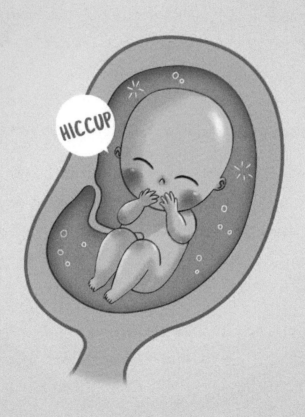

I have the hiccups

I am almost 2 inches tall and very active! I enjoy making fists with my hands and bending my elbows. I'm amazed at all the things I can do!

Something is happening inside of my mouth: the first buds of teeth are appearing. Whenever I open and close my mouth, I swallow some amniotic fluid. Something weird happened last time: I got a case of the hiccups. But it's not too bad, because I am glad that Mommy and Daddy are so happy. Grandma, Grandpa, and all of their friends now know that I am on my way.

I think that my Mommy is feeling great. She no longer feels nauseated as often as before.

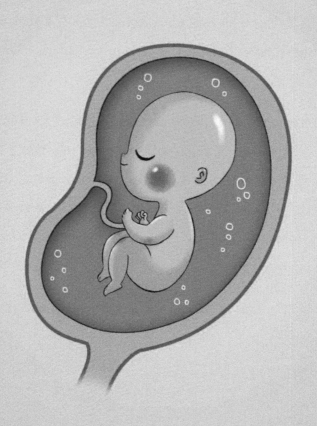

My bones are hardening

I am now almost 2.5 inches tall and weigh around 0.5 ounces. My bones were still very soft and gelatinous, but they are hardening now. My larynx and vocal cords continue to develop. I am sure I will have a beautiful voice one day.

Mommy and Daddy can watch my chest expand and contract on the ultrasound. It looks like I am breathing, but that is not the case. I still receive my oxygen through the umbilical cord, but practice makes perfect! It's useful to start practicing these respiratory movements early. Mommy's doctor says that this helps the development of my lungs.

Mommy is so excited that her tummy is starting to expand. Daddy thinks that her breasts have grown even larger. Mommy also started to crave some unusual food pairings.

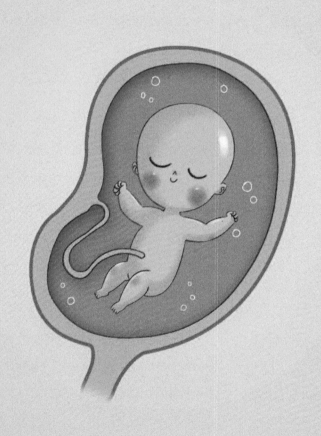

Mommy's belly is growing

I had a growth spurt last week, and I grew over half an inch! I am about 3 inches tall and weigh almost 0.9 ounces. I spend my days drinking amniotic fluid and kicking my arms and legs. The hiccups still bother me sometimes. They were even noticeable on the ultrasound.

Mommy's belly is getting rounder, but that's not just because of me. It is mainly due to the increased amount of amniotic fluid. Mommy has also gained a little weight. Her hormones are fluctuating right now, and she is not sleeping too well.

Mommy and Daddy often place their hands on her belly so that they can feel me. Unfortunately, this will not work out just yet. I am still too small to perform real "kicks", but I still enjoy it.

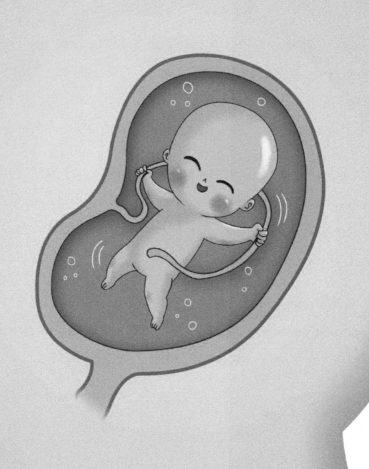

My reflexes are improving

You can watch me testing out my reflexes on the ultrasound. Mommy and Daddy were really excited when they saw that I reached for the umbilical cord with my tiny hands. It is so easy to make them happy! I can nod my head to my parents, and I can turn my head.

My eyes are fully developed, but they are still closed. Almost all of my organs are now working independently. I am 3.3 inches tall and weigh about 1.6 ounces. My Mommy is struggling with some mild swelling, but she says that this has some benefits. Her skin looks much smoother now.

The doctor is trying to figure out my sex again! I will not be able to hide it much longer, but I will try to fool him one last time.

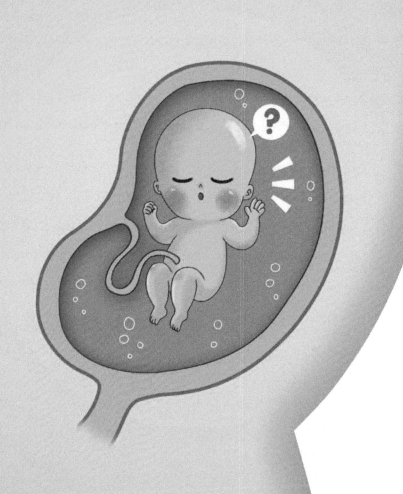

I can hear Mommy's voice

My ears have finally developed enough for me to hear sounds. The soft and rhythmic thumping must be Mommy's heartbeat. I like to listen to her heartbeat because it is so soothing. The thing I love the most is when Mommy and Daddy talk to me. I really like their voices. Mommy sometimes sings for me. Daddy tries to sing as well, but it is usually a bit off-key.

Oh, what was that humming noise? That must have been a car that just passed us by. The world is suddenly full of sounds! This is so exciting, and I am now sleeping a lot less and staying even more active.

By the way: I weigh over 2.5 ounces and am almost 4 inches tall. That is about the size of an apple!

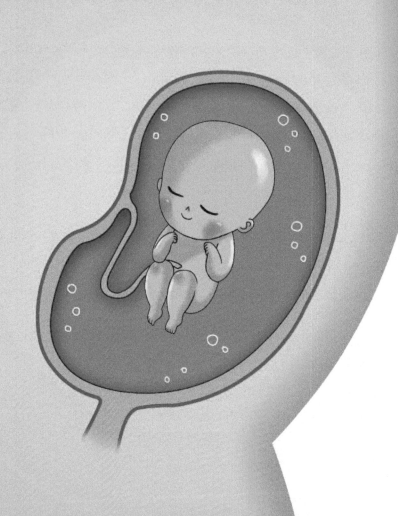

I am gaining some weight

Oh my, I am getting chubby! I am starting to gain some weight because I need a sufficient layer of fat to regulate my body temperature. Mommy is also gaining weight. If we keep going like this, the buttons of her pants might pop off. Maybe that is why she is looking for new clothes?

I weigh about 4 ounces and am over 4 inches tall. My hearing has improved significantly, and I can hear almost everything. I can even hear Mommy quietly farting! Unfortunately, some loud noises scare me a little. Those pesky hiccups keep bothering me.

My arms and legs continue to grow, and this changes the proportions of my body. My head does not look quite as large anymore.

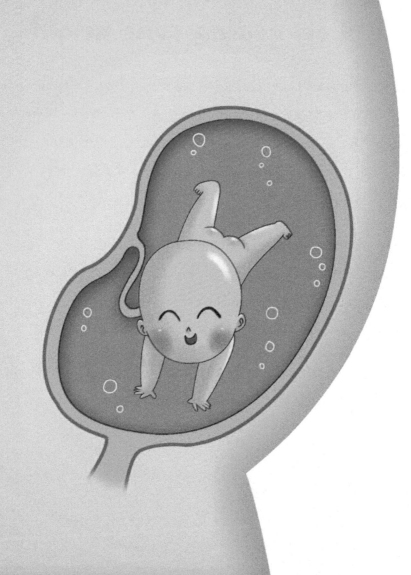

I keep exercising

I continue to kick my arms and legs and practice my water aerobics inside the amniotic sac. I am so big and strong that Mommy will soon be able to feel my movements.

All of this exercise makes me tired. I sleep about 20 hours each day, especially when Mommy is moving around. It feels as if she is rocking me to sleep.

Strangely, Mommy does not seem too happy about the fact that I like to be awake at night. Unfortunately, I still do not know the difference between daytime and nighttime. I am bored whenever she is not moving, and I have to keep busy somehow, right?

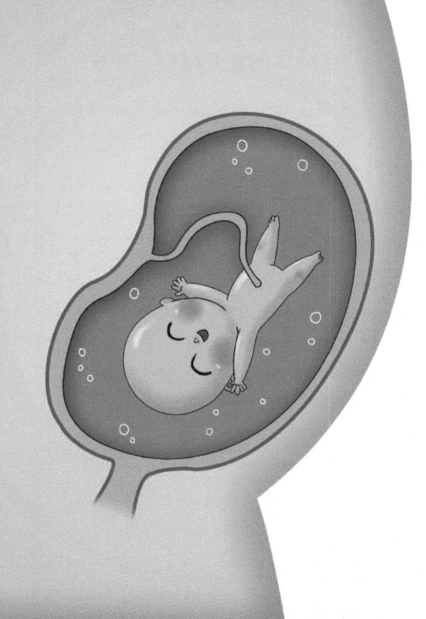

My heart is fully developed

The development of my heart is complete. It still beats twice as fast as the hearts of Mommy or Daddy. It pumps about 7 gallons of blood through my little body each day. That is pretty impressive, right?

I am over 5 inches tall and weigh 7 ounces. My intestines are starting to work. Mommy and Daddy are nervous because the second medical screening is coming up. I am looking forward to waving to my parents during the ultrasound. I think they will be impressed when they watch me do somersaults.

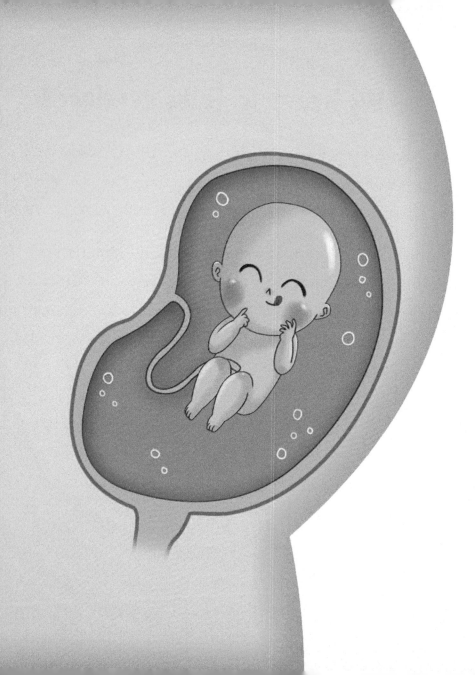

I have a sense of taste

Did you know that I have ten times more taste buds before I am born than afterward? This is why I can tell what Mommy has been eating whenever I taste the amniotic fluid. That is pretty cool! Please only eat delicious foods, Mommy!

My body hair is getting thicker. My workouts have also paid off. I am now so strong that Mommy can feel me moving around. Daddy can hear me when he places his ear on Mommy's belly. Hi, Daddy!

Mommy's belly cannot be concealed any longer. That is not surprising, because I now weigh around 8.5 ounces and am 5.5 inches tall!

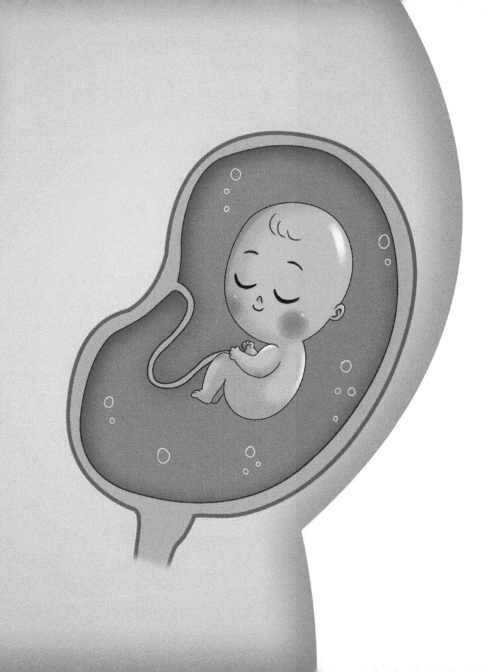

I am growing hair

The profile of my face is now more defined. My eyebrows, eyelashes, and hair have begun to grow. My facial expressions are much more alive. I can raise my eyebrows skeptically whenever I do not like something. Mommy does that all the time. I don't think I will need to raise my eyebrows too often because I am content most of the time.

I weigh 10.5 ounces and am almost 10 inches tall. I have grown a lot in just one week! Aside from kicking my arms and legs, my favorite activity is sleeping. A consistent sleep-wake cycle has been established by now.

I have also discovered my favorite sleeping position! Mommy can feel my movements whenever I am awake.

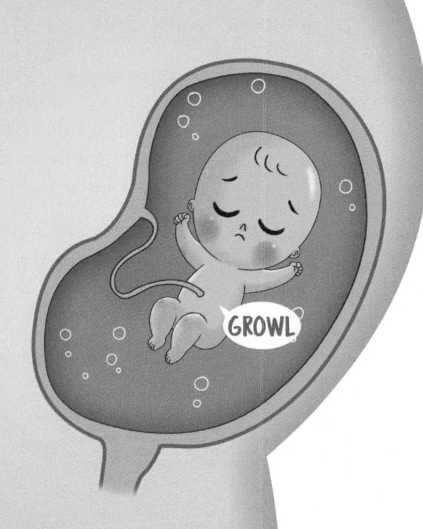

I need lots of energy

I look like a miniature version of a fully developed baby by now. All parts are there, and my motor skills are excellent. Mommy can definitely feel that whenever she tries to lie down. My hair, eyebrows, and eyelashes are a bit pale and could use a little more color.

Since I am practically fully developed, my next goal is to gain lots of weight. That is why Mommy often feels ravenously hungry. I am very hungry as well!

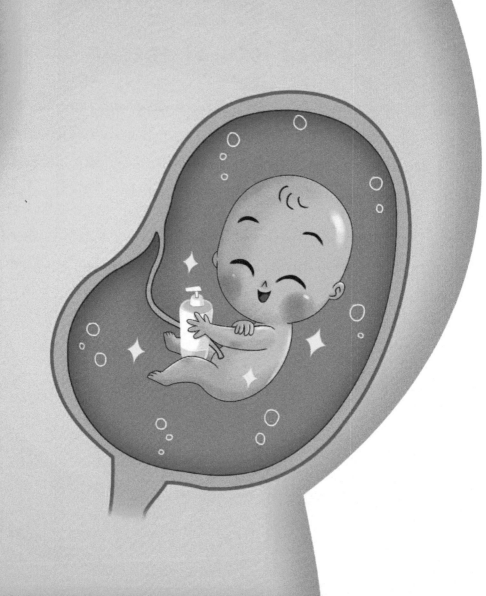

I have been moisturizing

The sebaceous glands next to the hair follicles that cover my body have been busy with the production of the so-called vernix. It covers me from head to toe. The vernix acts as a moisturizer, and it keeps my skin soft while I am floating in the amniotic fluid. I still cannot see anything, but you can see my eyes moving underneath my eyelids in the ultrasound.

Mommy's belly is nice and round by now. Her old dresses and pants do not fit anymore. She sometimes feels a little bit dizzy because my presence has caused an increase in her body's blood volume. That is not dangerous for me because my circulatory system works independently, but it can bother Mommy.

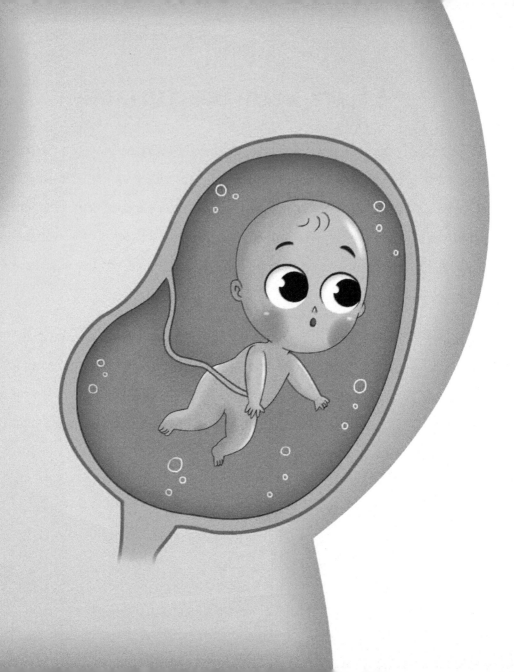

I will take a look around

My taste buds are now fully developed. I love sweets! No wonder that Mommy craves chocolate these days. Mommy and I continue to gain weight together. Somehow, Daddy is gaining weight, too. I wonder if a baby is growing inside Daddy's tummy as well because his belly is getting rounder...

I weigh 19 ounces and am 11.4 inches tall. I can even sit up inside Mommy's belly. My bones keep my body nice and stable. Things feel a lot more cramped inside my little home so I started to open my eyes to take a look around.

I still have enough room to play and exercise, but I wonder how much longer this will last? My lungs are growing steadily. I am happy about that because I want to greet my parents with a loud scream.

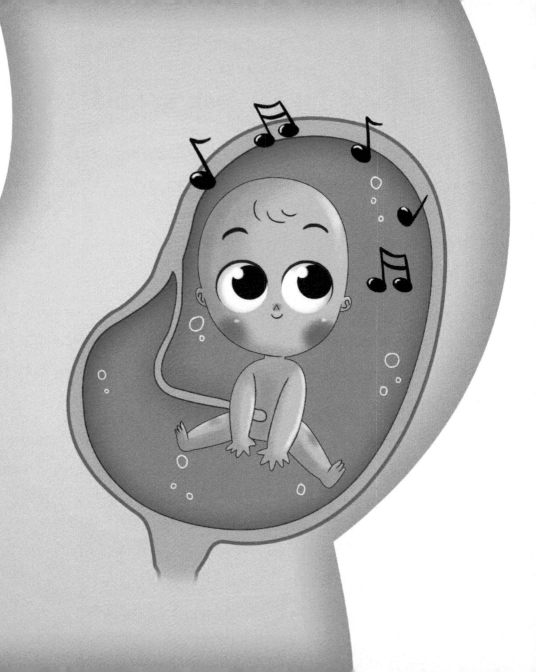

My perception is improving

I notice everything: every sound, every jolt, and every voice. That was fun at first, but it is starting to get on my nerves every once in a while. When I do not like something, it shows. My pulse becomes more rapid and I move around more hectically. Mommy and Daddy will talk to me, and that makes me happy. I can remember their voices, and I am able to distinguish them from all the other voices in the world.

I am practicing how to sit up inside of Mommy's belly. It is working much better now that my sense of equilibrium is developing. I am changing on the outside as well. I was a pretty wrinkly creature, but my skin is much smoother now. The increased blood flow to my skin gives me a rosy complexion. My weight gain is finally paying off, and I am becoming more and more beautiful every day.

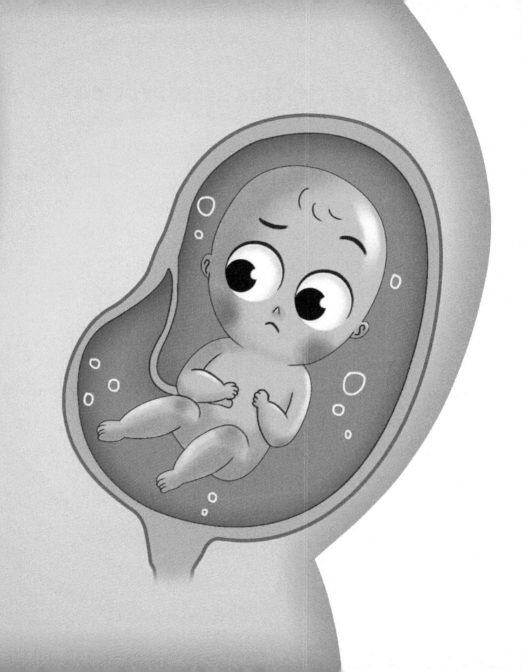

I have less and less room

I suspected that this might happen, and I can definitely feel it now. The bigger I get, the less room I have to play. I can feel the boundaries of my apartment.

Have I really grown this much? I certainly have: I weigh a little over 28 ounces, and I am 12.5 inches tall. Since I am so big, I take up a lot of room in Mommy's belly. I think that I accidentally push on her bladder sometimes and that I often interfere with her digestion...I am sorry, Mommy!

I can tell the difference between light and dark. The light sometimes affects my sleep, but I just blink and turn my back to it.

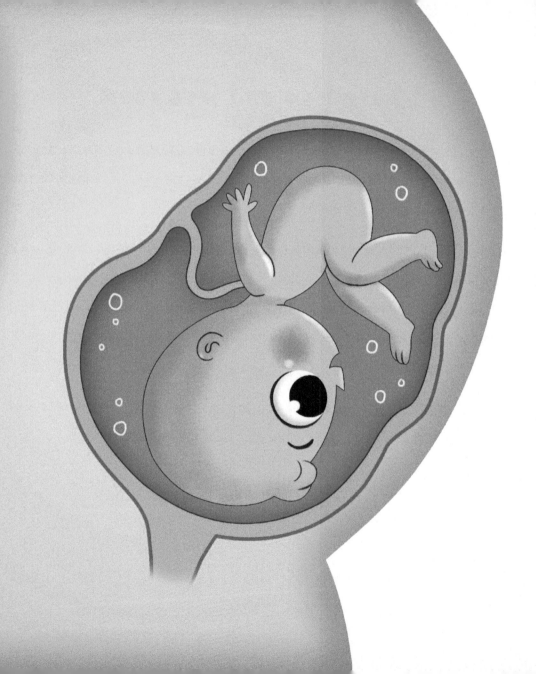

I am kicking around

I use whatever space I have left. Mommy is amazed that she can sometimes feel my little feet in her lower abdomen in the morning, but then they are close to her ribs in the evening — or vice versa. Daddy can also feel me when he places his hand on Mommy's belly.

My organs are fully matured and functional, except for my lungs. But there's no rush. I weigh over 2.2 lbs. and am about 13 inches long.

Mommy struggles with fluid retention. Fluid is a problem in general because my weight puts a lot of pressure on her bladder. I cannot help it! If my apartment would only expand a little bit more...

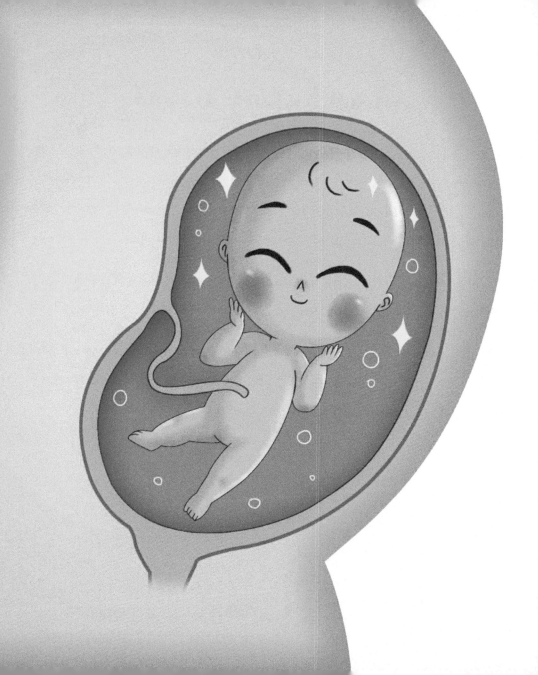

I open and close my eyes

I do the same thing the adults do: I close my eyes when I go to sleep, and I open them when I wake up. My vision is not quite perfect, but it does not have to be as long as I am in Mommy's belly. Everything looks pretty much the same around here anyway.

My face is fully developed — individual, unmistakable, and especially attractive! The color of my eyes is not certain just yet. It might even change after I am born. Mommy and Daddy got a good look at my face during the 3D ultrasound. I am now over 14 inches tall and weigh 2.4 lbs.

I think that my apartment is changing. I hope I will finally have more space. Maybe not. The top of my apartment is thickening, and the bottom is long and round. That's not quite what I had envisioned, but I am excited to find out what is going to happen next.

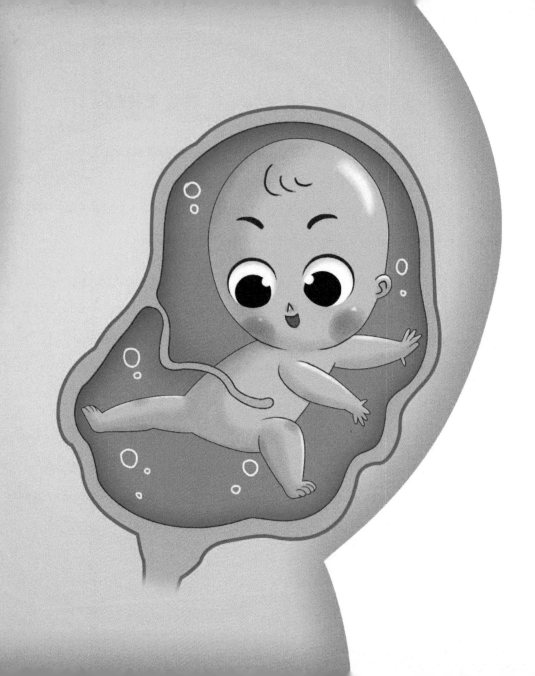

I am producing antibodies

I heard that life "outside" can be really challenging for my small body. I am relieved that I am getting antibodies through the placenta. They will protect me from several illnesses. My immune system is preparing for the time after birth. Luckily, we still have lots of time.

I am 14.6 inches tall and weigh almost 2.9 lbs. I can regulate my body temperature all by myself now. Everything is going well so far, but it is terribly cramped in here! I cannot kick my legs too well anymore, but I often elbow my Mommy in the stomach.

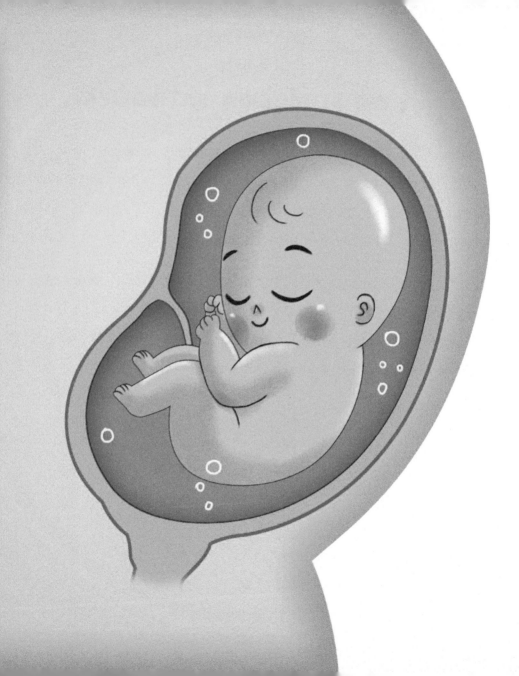

I need to change positions

Oops, my fine hair is falling out! I was covered with this coat of soft hair all this time, but I guess I no longer need it. The hair on my head is growing quickly. I wonder what my hair color will be?

I gained 0.2 lbs., and I currently weigh 3.1 lbs. I am pretty chunky, aren't I? My bones are stronger, and my skin is much smoother. I definitely cannot roughhouse in here any longer. I am almost uncomfortable, and I had to assume a new position. I press my chin to my chest and pull my arms and legs close to my body. Now I am at least somewhat comfortable, but I think I will eventually get tired of this small apartment if this continues!

Mommy also cannot move as much as she used to. Her belly has grown to a pretty impressive size.

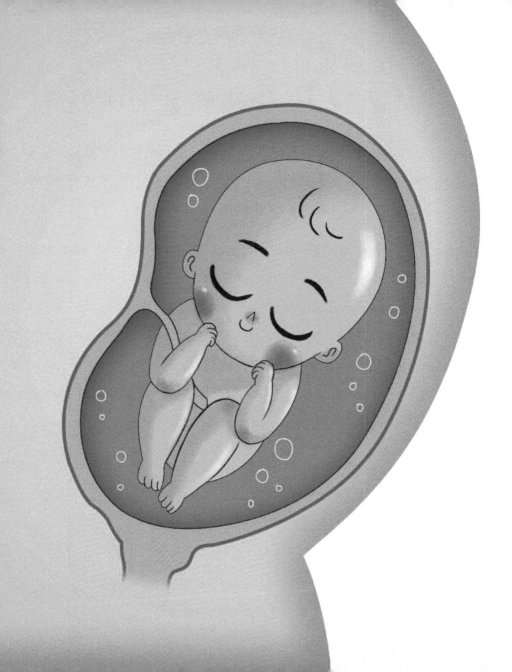

My senses are fully developed

I can see, feel, smell, hear and taste. The majority of my development is complete. The last weeks have been exhausting, and I am not even getting paid for all my hard work! It's time to get some rest.

Mommy and Daddy are starting to think about the delivery and the time after I am born. Mommy thinks that many things that she used to be able to do with ease are much more difficult now. She should not complain this much. I am also going through a lot in here!

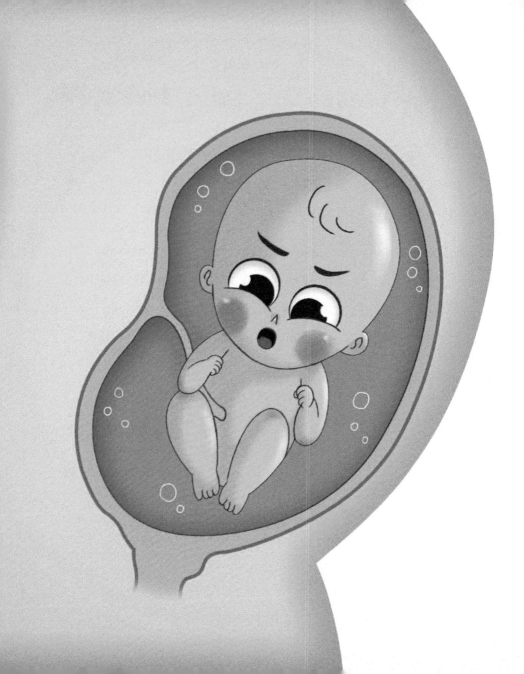

I am practicing my breathing

I am practicing inhalations and exhalations in the amniotic fluid. You never know when you might need those skills! My lungs will be fully developed soon.

I sometimes swallow some amniotic fluid during these breathing exercises. Since I am so big and strong, Mommy can really feel my hiccups. I am also extremely hungry and need a lot of nutrients so that I can gain weight and grow even more. I hope Mommy continues to eat as much as she does right now!

I currently weigh 4 lbs. and am 16 inches tall.

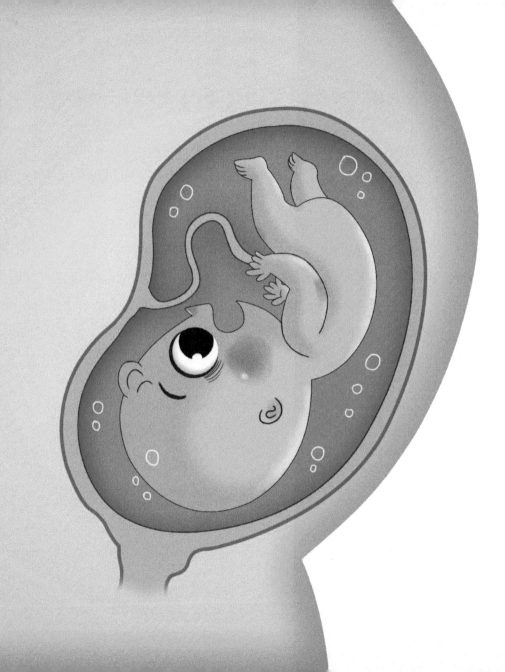

I am doing a headstand

I just wanted to move around a little bit, but suddenly I was upside down. Mommy felt a slight tug in her belly. I cannot sit upright anymore. Oh well, I will just stay like this.

Nothing surprises me anymore, but there is not much left for me to do other than to grow and gain more weight. I spend most of my time sleeping. Mommy has been able to breathe better after I did my headstand. I think that this was a good move for both of us.

Mommy and Daddy often talk to me. I am looking forward to finally seeing them. I have a feeling that I will not have to wait much longer.

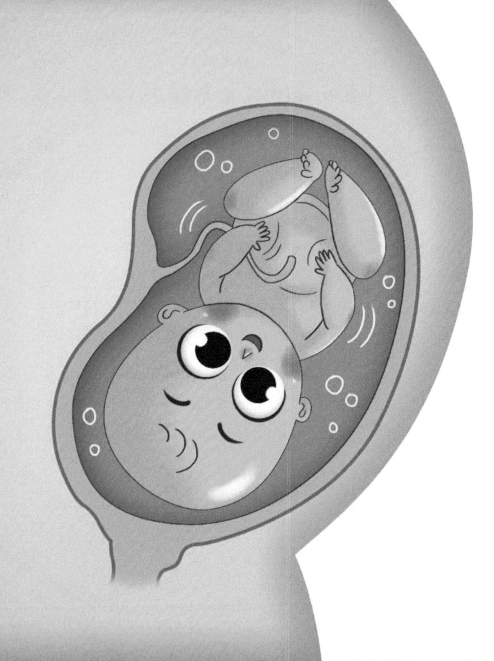

The final touches

I am fully developed and would do just fine outside of Mommy's belly. Although it is not as comfortable as before, I still want to stay in here just a little bit longer. At least I do not have to worry about anything as long as I am in here because Mommy takes great care of me. It's like an "all-inclusive hotel".

I am over 17 inches tall and weigh 4.9 lbs. It is hard to believe that I was a tiny speck just a few weeks ago. My fingernails are still very soft, but they now extend past my fingertips.

Mommy thinks that I am pretty heavy. Well, that is her own fault because she keeps feeding me! Luckily, she doesn't have to go back to work this week and will get a chance to relax. Mommy and Daddy are preparing everything for my arrival. When will they roll out the red carpet? A star like me deserves a grand welcome!

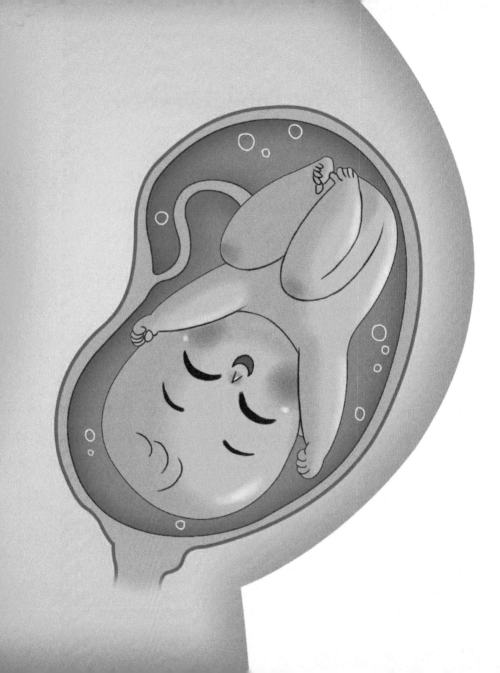

Preparing for delivery

Mommy can feel mild contractions every once in a while. Those are not real contractions, but Mommy still gets really excited because she thinks that it is time. Well, she can forget about that for now! I decided to take my time before I make my way into the world. I am feeling well and have everything I need in here.

I gained more than 0.6 lbs. this week! I now weigh 5.5 lbs. Mommy's belly is humungous! Unfortunately, she has not been able to sleep or bend over too well. I do feel a little sorry for her.

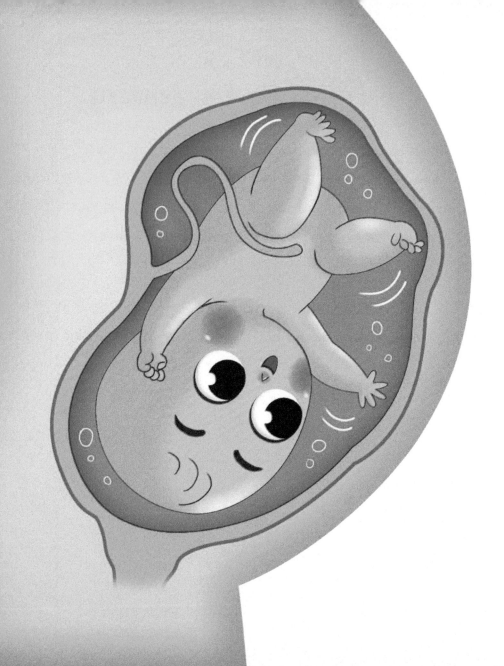

I am thriving

I am now 18 inches tall. Since I am tucking my arms and legs in, I am about the size of a honeydew melon! No wonder that Mommy says that many activities are exhausting for her. Who would want to carry a melon around all day?

I look like a "complete" baby in the ultrasound. Since Mommy's belly does not have much more room for me, my hands and feet look like little bumps under her skin whenever I push against her belly. That seems to make her happy, so I keep doing it.

She can see where I am, and Daddy is also fascinated by this. Sometimes they disagree about whether they have spotted a hand or a foot.

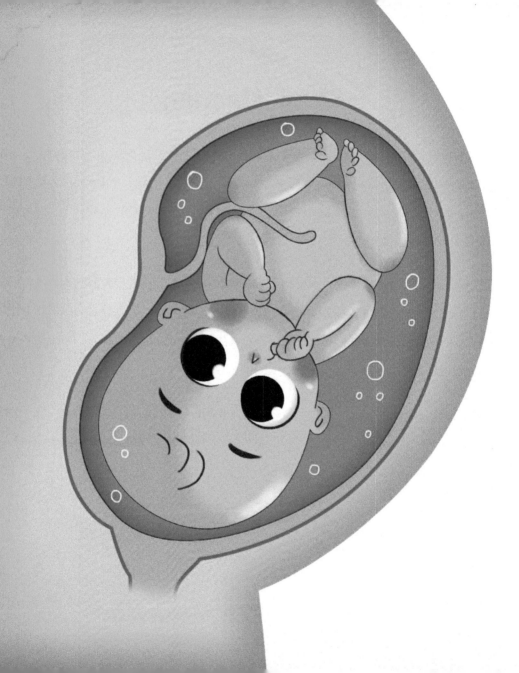

Waiting, waiting, waiting

I sleep and dream. What else is there to do? There is not much to entertain me in here. I have not had enough room to play for a while now. The only thing I can still do is suck on my thumb.

Mommy is feeling sluggish. If I decided to leave now, I would still be a bit early – but I would be perfectly fine! However, I am not ready to leave yet. I will just trust my instincts. I will feel when the time is right.

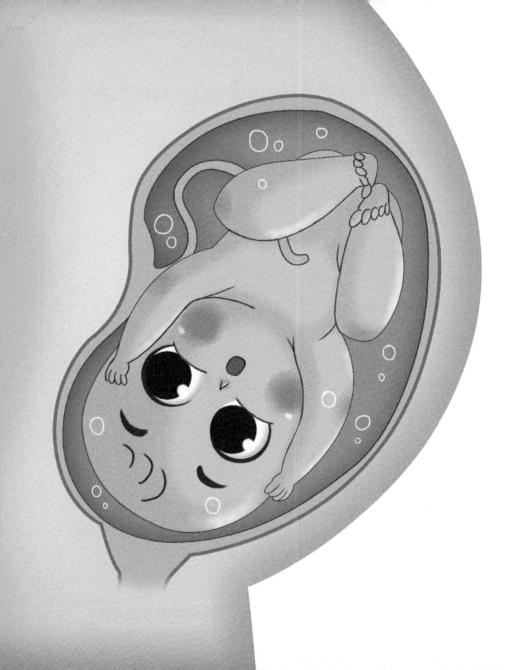

The final stretch

If I was born today, I would not be a preemie anymore. I am 19 inches tall and weigh 6.8 lbs.

I think that my time in Mommy's belly is almost up. I have assumed my birthing position. My head is lodged in Mommy's pelvis. The false labor pains that used to alarm Mommy have stopped.

My parents are excited and nervous, just like me! I will have to leave my home. I wonder what will await me outside? I heard that the great care I have received in the "Hotel Mommy" will continue out there for 18 more years!

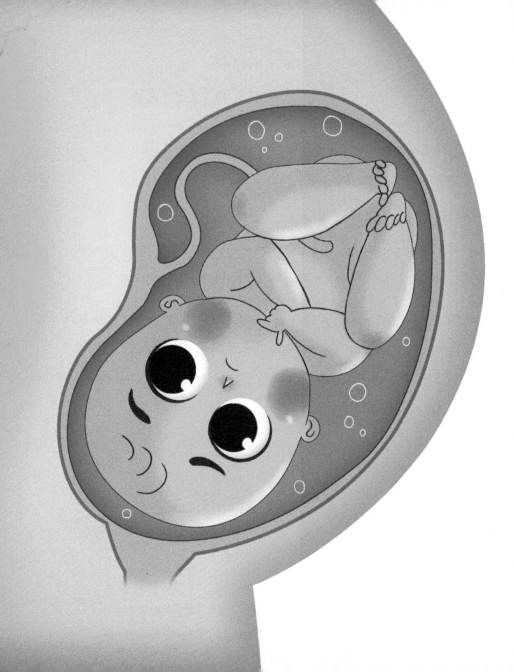

There is no more room!

My once comfortable home is not so cozy anymore. I have no more room and keep bumping into things. Unlike a few weeks ago, I am now very calm and barely move.

The vernix that has been protecting my skin is getting thinner, and not much of the soft hair is left. I guess I will not need these protective features any longer. I am ready for life outside of Mommy's belly. Do I really have to leave already? I am not a coward, but I am a bit nervous. I am still undecided. Maybe I should spend a few more days in here to gain some weight and grow a little more. Just to be safe!

Nonetheless, I guess it is about time to say goodbye to my fancy apartment.

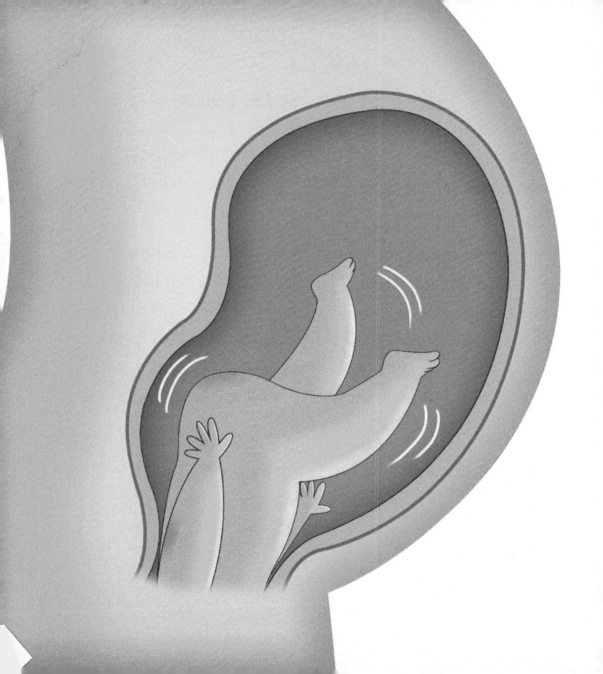

It is time!

I have reached my birth weight! I weigh 7.7 lbs. Mommy is uncomfortable most of the time, so I have decided to come out now.

The cramped conditions in her belly are really bothering me now, too. The oxygen and amniotic fluid are running out. I also want to finally find out what Mommy and Daddy look like. However, Mommy and I need to put in a lot of effort before I can meet them. Nobody told me how hard my head has to work during the birthing process! Daddy turned quite pale although he is not doing anything at all.

Mommy pushes a lot, and it seems like everything is getting tighter. Oh, what is that? I am slowly being pushed out of my home, and suddenly everything is very bright!

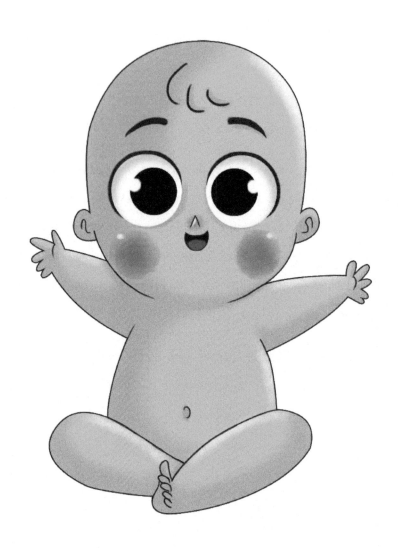

We did it!

Hooray! I made my way into this world, and Mommy is cradling me in her arms. Being born was really exhausting, and I still need to get used to the world.

It was 98.6 degrees inside Mommy's belly, but it is much colder and brighter outside. I also got to meet a lot of new people. It took some time to adjust to all of these changes. I could finally hear my own voice! As soon as I was born, I tested my lungs. The strange man in the white coat said that they are very strong.

Mommy and I are very tired, and we need to recover. Daddy is also exhausted, but he is very happy. I am looking forward to spending time with my parents. I am sure that I will keep them busy!

Thank you!

You have arrived at the end of this book! I want to take a moment to thank you for reading!

Did you enjoy this little book about pregnancy, and did it make you smile? If so, I would appreciate it if you took two minutes to review it on Amazon. Reviews from readers are helpful feedback for us authors, and they can help other customers decide whether to purchase this book.

I want to thank you for your time and effort, and I wish you and your child all the best and lots of joy and happiness.

You are wonderful!

Made in the USA
Columbia, SC
19 December 2021

51990152R00050